Making Rounds

IIt's amazing what you see,
what you don't want to see,
and how you start to
see everything different
the moment you start

KJ Jackson, Lpn

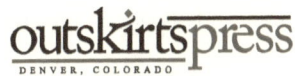

The opinions expressed in this manuscript are solely the opinions of the author and do not represent the opinions or thoughts of the publisher. The author has represented and warranted full ownership and/or legal right to publish all the materials in this book.

Making Rounds
It's amazing what you see, what you don't want to see,
and how you start to see everything different the moment you start
All Rights Reserved.
Copyright © 2016 KJ Jackson, Lpn
v3.0

Writing Services: K. Martinez
Author Photo: Manuelle Whitfield
Cover © 2016 Multimedia Vidjewelz. All rights reserved - used with permission.

This book may not be reproduced, transmitted, or stored in whole or in part by any means, including graphic, electronic, or mechanical without the express written consent of the publisher except in the case of brief quotations embodied in critical articles and reviews.

Outskirts Press, Inc.
http://www.outskirtspress.com

ISBN: 978-1-4787-7508-9

Outskirts Press and the "OP" logo are trademarks belonging to Outskirts Press, Inc.

PRINTED IN THE UNITED STATES OF AMERICA

For: My mother, Anna:
There is no love like that of a mother. Your undying love will forever live inside of me.

For: My sister, Lieutenant Lauren Carthan: You are the toughest soldier I know, on and off of the battlefield. Thank you for always believing in me, even when I doubted myself.

To: My son, Darren (Jashawn):
My greatest love. My true inspiration. My biggest fan. My motivation. May your dreams take you on a journey that reaches far beyond the skies and miles past the moon. Everything you want in life is already yours . . . go and get it, son.
Love, Mommy Wow

Table of Contents

Prologue i
Code Blue 1
Everybody's Favorite 5
You Make the Call 8
In God We Trust 15
A Lesson to Learn 21
Politics in Nursing 26
My Crew 30
911 to 119 35
And So It Was 40
Grapes of Wrath 45
Missed Diagnosis 53
Epilogue 59
Acknowledgements 62

Memoir: Before I open up and share my dream and pieces of my life with you, I can not and will not pass up the opportunity to share a memory of me as a child playing nurse.

I was about ten years old when I saw my eight year olds cousin Clay performing daredevil stunts on his dirt bike. Although he had no formal training in performing these stunts he continued to attempt them nonetheless. I watched him and his brother Colin as they made a large ramp of plywood and bricks piled high off the ground so they could elevate into the air as they pedaled to gain speed. The whole idea looked dangerous to me, but I can't say that I was surprised. In fact, nothing that my cousins did surprised me. They were both fearless.

As Clay attempted to try one more time to elevate higher than before jumping over the ramp, he somehow managed to lose control of the bike and was thrown into the air, landing on his right knee in what appeared to be a pothole. As I ran to his rescue, I could see the oversized gash in his knee filled with rocks and debris as blood rushed out racing down his leg. "Do something Lexi, do something !", Clay yelled. Lexi was my childhood nickname short for Alexis, my middle name. Again, I was ten years old, I had no idea what to do. As his brother and I helped him into the house, into the bathroom, I poured cup after cup of water directly into the wound trying to remove the debris. As I drowned out his crying as best as I could, I reached for the roll of toilet paper and began packing every inch of the open wound. Wherever there was a drop of blood, I packed it until every drop was absorbed. Finally, I covered it with paper towels and applied scotch tape to hold it in place. Everything seemed back to normal. He was happy, I was happy. I was a hero in his eyes. Needless to say as soon as our parents came home he was taken to the emergency room where he received eight stitches after a very painful debridement..

Let's face it, you don't have to be a medical professional to know that the nursing care I performed was the epitome of poor nursing despite my intentions to be a good samaritan and a good big cousin. Nonetheless, for the record, I would like to acknowledge that my cousin Clay, was my first unofficial patient .

Prologue

It all started late one night in the midst of a deep, dark December when I fell asleep and had a dream, a dream fascinating enough that I felt compelled to write a book to tell the world my adventures of this dream. I dreamt I was a veteran nurse of fifteen years. I dreamt I had coworkers and I worked in the confines of a prestigious hospital in Chicago. I dreamt that I faced some of the most difficult challenges of my life. It was during this dream that I embarked on a journey down a path that may have been much more than just another ordinary road. Throughout this dream, I tell the story of each road I traveled and each experience and lesson that came from it all. Well . . . almost all of it. The last chapter of the dream may forever remain a mystery . . .

....

Who am I? I am KJ.

For those who know me, know I am most credited for being a fixer of all things. If something is broken, I'm called in to fix it, long before it ever becomes a problem.

I command and demand order.

I put things in order and I keep things in order. I am a gift to those whose supervision I work under, and a drill sergeant to those that work under me. Many people applaud me for my laid back, calm demeanor in a crisis-like situation. If chaos erupts, such as a Code Blue or any type of nursing crisis, I am the nurse MOST nurses want by their side to assist and take the lead in the situation. I have a natural knack for teaching others.

As ironic as it may sound, being a nurse was never really my dream; my dream was becoming a teacher. Essentially, I have successfully combined the two professions into one. I sincerely enjoy teaching both rookie nurses and seasoned nurses anything and everything that I can teach them. Even the most successful nurses in my hospital humble themselves to ask for my nursing opinions in any given situation.

I am an aggressive supervisor, a quick thinker, and a team leader for my peers; however, I am also a team player, and I have made many sacrifices in my career for the benefit of my team.

I am a valuable resource. Once, I even memorized a company's handbook of corporate policies and I could get anybody out of any situation and save their job. I've even saved myself a few times, sure enough. I've been told that there are some strong attorney qualities within my personality.

Am I cocky, as some would accuse me of being? Nope! Confident. Get it right!

Am I an Ass ? (as I've been called so many times) Nope! I am assured, but you got the first three letters right!

In other words, I am bold enough to say what other people think but are too timid to say themselves.

I don't prey on the weak. I challenge the strong; it sends a louder message. For instance, I choose not to reprimand a staff of nursing assistants because the unit is a mess. Instead, I choose to confront the nurses in front of the CNAs and ask them why have they allowed the CNAs to shame them and have the unit in shambles.

I remain PROFESSIONAL at all times. No matter what the situation is, I am ALWAYS 100 percent professional.

I'm good at what I do. Even those that dislike me refuse to discredit me or my talents. Everyone I've ever worked with—nurses, CNAs, nurse managers, administrators, and hospital chief clinical officers—call me KJ. Nooooooobody anywhere calls me Kerrin, ever! Those two letters when said together in that order, says, "ORDER, ORDER IN THE COURT." People either love me or they hate me; there is no in between and there never will be.

Who am I, you ask? I am me . . .

I am KJ.

Code Blue

I can remember it vividly, like it was only yesterday. It was a beautiful autumn day and there was a bright, sunny October sky. I remember that a strong feeling of euphoria and utter happiness swept over me as I finished orientation that afternoon. All of my schooling and subsequent training was officially over, and I was finally ready to begin my career as a charge nurse. To begin the day, there was a list of tasks I needed to complete in chronological order. In addition to completing my tasks, I was also responsible for overseeing a motivated team of Certified Nursing Assistants and supervising the completion of their assignments. For me, passing the exams had been simple. Grasping a full and thorough understanding of the medication administration record was as simple as 1-2-3. It seemed as if this was too good to be true. The pay was pretty well, too—$16.00 dollars per hour in 1993 was just as good as it sounds. After all, I'd spent the last five years working at Sears, twice as hard, earning a whopping $6.75 per hour! Feeling a strong sense of pride in myself and fixated on my monumental accomplishment, I thought to myself, "It's funny how life works out like that!"

As I was smiling from ear to ear, enjoying my first day in my new role, one of the CNAs approached me with a small piece of paper with a patient's vital signs scribbled within its content. The vital signs showed the following: 72/47, 42, 10, 96 degrees. Anyone who has any working knowledge of nursing would know these vital signs are NOT GOOD! In a flush of sheer panic, my mind immediately began racing to the worst possible situation. At that precise moment, my head was spinning and I feared the worst, although I was praying for the best. Doing my best to keep calm under the severe circumstances I had found myself in, the logical and analytical module of my mind raced back to every textbook page I've ever read about abnormal vital signs. I thought to myself, "If I only had my damn med surg' book now . . . damn it! I'm a nurse; I'm supposed to know these things! What do I do?!"

Trying my best to appear calm in the face of panic, I casually walked to the patient's room, hoping and praying he was still alive. As I approached him I could see he looked quite abnormal. His bones were frail, his body was cold as ice, and all the extremities suddenly came alive. Faced with the surreal possibility that this man could be dying right in front of my very eyes I silently screamed to myself, "What did the book say to do? Come on, Kerrin! Try to remember! What did the book say to do?!?!" Suddenly, I drew a blank.

Paralyzed with fear, I can recall feeling light headed, as if I was going to faint, as I ran to the nurse that had mentored me; I frantically asked her if she could talk me through this debilitating scenario. I screamed, "Oh, my god! Beverly, please help me! This man is turning blue before my eyes. His vital signs are abnormal and I do not know what to do!"

I was sweating. I was trembling. My face was flushed, as if I had seen a ghost. With my heart racing and my throat narrowly caving in, I knew there was no turning back from this moment. Although I had learned CPR in nursing school, I had never been exposed to a dying person before, and given the intense fear of the situation, I quite honestly didn't think that I would be able to cope with it. I felt as if I was going to be swept away by my emotions at any moment.

Suddenly, in the most calming voice I've ever heard, the nurse said to me, "Well, Kerrin, brace yourself. All of that is about to change. If the doctor does not call you back be prepared to call a Code Blue."

"Code what?," I said. It's now becoming evident that I missed more days of clinicals than I'd ever thought before. I kept frantically thinking, "What is a Code Blue? What do I do first?" Running out of options, I felt weak and defeated. I felt as if I wanted to crawl in a hole and cry. I was terrified, not only for the dying man, but for my career as well. My anxious mind continued to race with intrusive thoughts and a strong fear of impending doom rapidly coming my way.

As we walked into room 301, time meant nothing to me. Although the walk to the room was only a mere couple of seconds, it felt like a lifetime of walking before we finally arrived in the room. As the patient and I made eye contact, I could see that he was barely breathing. His non-rebreather oxygen mask was delivering 15 liters of oxygen; however, he was still turning blue at a rapid pace.

At that moment in time, I can recall hearing an overhead page. "Kerrin, you have Dr. Khahdrid holding on line one. Kerrin, Dr. Khahdrid on line one."

The sound of that page rang through the hospital's hallways like a song from the Lord. I can remember screaming, "Yes, yes, thank you, Jesus!"

In the nick of time, the doctor ordered me to send the patient out 911. As the ambulance arrived at the hospital, the patient was still barely breathing, yet he was still hanging on for his life, still fighting to survive. Although he was still breathing and sparsely holding on, his pulse was barely palpable. As they transferred his near-lifeless body to the ambulance stretcher, I can vividly remember closing my eyes, folding my hands, and saying a silent prayer to the Lord. I remember shedding a tear, thinking that if this man didn't make it, I'm not sure I would be able to live with myself. I remember thinking of his friends, his family, and wondering how they would all react if this man didn't make it. Right there outside the hospital, I remember asking God for two important things. First, I asked God to forgive me for being negligent, for not being as prepared as I should have been, for not being as equipped as I needed to be to save this poor man's life. I then said a prayer for this man and his family, asking God to take care of him. I also prayed that this man would forgive me for not knowing what to do if he made it out of this predicament alive.

The paramedics then began performing chest compressions as they rolled the patient to the elevator. Still praying to the Lord above, I prayed that I would be given the strength to forgive myself for failing my first real-world test. I prayed I would be strong enough to put this unfortunate situation behind and be able to successfully move forward in my career and in my life after this. In that instance, I can remember immediately thinking of other careers I could have (and probably should have) considered. I can recall how foolish my thoughts were just less than an hour ago. My thoughts had been that this job was going to be easy, a cakewalk. What was I thinking? It was my very first real world test, and the word "easy" was nowhere to be found.

At that very moment, I knew that my profession was much more than just an average nine-to-five job. I knew I was responsible for people's lives. In that very instance, I remember opening my eyes, staring into the sky where I had just prayed to God, and I remember thinking, "Lesson one learned. I wonder what is in store for lesson two? Lord, please help me through this!"

Everybody's Favorite

After five long, fulfilling years of nursing, I am undoubtedly not the same person I was when I first began my career just five years prior. I am a different person, and certainly a different nurse as well. I am assertive, aggressive, and I have learned the fine art of multitasking, which is not an area I was proficient in before. These are the core fundamentals needed for nursing that you simply cannot learn in nursing school and multitasking is one of them.

Being able to be aggressive and assertive is critical to really being able to survive in this field. I can recall having a conversation with one of my colleagues, another nurse on my team. She said to me, "The reason CNAs don't like to work with you is because you are too hard on them. You are always riding them. They don't make much and you expect them to work, work, work!" I could not believe what I was hearing. After a couple of minutes I could see that her lips were still moving, which let me know she was still talking; however, I couldn't hear anything else she said. Angry and in disbelief by what I was hearing, I had successfully managed to completely tune her out. Sitting there, growing angrier with each passing second, I could no longer hold in my feelings.

Finally, after becoming more and more frustrated, I mustered up the courage and said to her, "The reason the CNAs enjoy working with you is because you allow them to do absolutely nothing. Their first set of rounds and their last set of rounds are all in one. You allow them to let the residents saturate in their own urine all night while the staff sleeps. One hour after the shifts begins everyone on your floor is eating and gossiping. And of course, everybody knows how much productivity will drastically decrease when stomachs are full."

This is one of the many classic examples I've faced throughout my career where I've had to stand up for myself and take charge when the time called for it; otherwise, I would not be the nurse that I am today. I am outspoken, and I do not allow anyone to criticize myself or my work in a destructive manner. I'm open to criticism as long as it is constructive and it is delivered with professionalism.

It's 6 a.m., one hour and a half before my shift ends. The echoed whining of the residents who don't want to be awakened is quickly silenced by an amplified voice screaming, "Code Blue Room 139, Code Blue Room 139!" In a matter of just seconds, every nurse, every CNA, everybody who is anybody makes a mad dash directly to the location of the shouting. By the time I had arrived, I saw three nurses frantically performing Cardiopulmonary Resuscitation on a man lying on the floor, not moving. The patient's fists were tightly clenched and both arms were extended in front of him with his elbows bent. The same position applied to his legs as well. His knees were bent and made the shape of a perfect right angle. I shouted, "What the hell?!" For whatever reason, my question went answered.

It took about five minutes before 911 arrived, although each passing second felt like a lifetime because of the immense level of fear that was instilled in each and every one of us. Everyone was in panic mode and very worried that this man may not make it out alive. When the emergency team made their way to the scene, it took a mere three seconds before the fire chief yelled out, "Discontinue CPR. This patient has been dead for about eight or nine hours!" Shaken by the news I had just heard, I was completely speechless. My head was full of questions, but I couldn't get myself to say anything at the time. Frightened, the staff just sat there in utter disbelief by the news they had just received. It was official; the man was dead.

As if the tragic event itself wasn't enough, it was the very next day that I read a statement from a different CNA who was also on duty when the event occurred . The CNA, Marilyn, stated that at the start of the shift the patient was sitting in his chair asleep. Because this was a patient who frequently fell and had a diagnosis of dementia, the assigned CNA didn't bother to turn the patient's light off and put him to bed. Instead, the CNA allowed him to sleep in the chair he sat in. Furthermore, the CNA, Marilyn also reported that when the assigned CNA did her next three sets of rounds the patient still sat in the chair asleep. It wasn't until 6 a.m., when the nurse went into the patient's room to do a scheduled accucheck check that the nurse realized that the man sitting in the chair wasn't asleep; he was dead. Seeing and hearing these kinds of things changes you. You are no longer the same person. Your attitude and perception of the entire world changes. You, essentially, become a different person simply because you have a more profound appreciation as well as understanding of life and just how fragile it is. Tomorrow is promised to no one, and no one is an exception to this rule.

You Make the Call

Somewhere in the midst of ending my career as a rookie nurse to becoming the seasoned, professional nurse that I am today, I truly discovered what it meant to be in charge and function as a charge nurse. Being a charge nurse can be as intense as ever, and trust me, I've had countless experiences that have made me realize just how tough the position can be. When you're a charge nurse, there's never a dull moment, and there is always an emergency that needs to be catered to. This is especially true for the 7 a.m. to 3 p.m. shift.

The 7 a.m. to 3 p.m. shift is a shift unlike any of the others. Most days are filled endlessly with tedious task. There are so many people to answer to, and everyone has seemingly endless demands as compared to other shifts. To break down some of the stress of the shift, I would often challenge another nurse by racing to complete a morning medicine pass. Let me just say that as competitive as I am and as much as I love to win, I would *never* challenge a nurse that I question may not *already* be passing their medications out as they should. The last thing that a half-assed nurse needs is a reason to be half of the half-assed that they already are. I know that may come off as arrogant or cocky, but trust me, there are those kinds of nurses employed in the nursing profession. Some of you are reading this book hoping I don't start calling names.

I often wondered how part-time or PRN nurses (nurses called only when needed) could finish a two-hour medicine pass in forty-five minutes or less. Mind you, they seldom know the patients or their regularly scheduled meds. I, however, could be the regular nurse for a unit five days a week, have their medications memorized, and still could not complete this task in less than an hour and a half. Therefore, the mere idea of completing this task in thirty to forty-five minutes is simply impossible! While I'm not accusing them of not passing out their meds, I am simply saying that a two-hour med pass minus thirty minutes of labor simply does not equal a complete medication pass.

You do the math. Better yet, let's all do the math:

40 patients require medications. It takes approximately 2 hours to administer them all. The average patient requires approximately 3 minutes of the nurse's attention. If the nurse has completed her entire med pass in 30 minutes, they have either passed meds at a rate of 42 seconds per patient, or only 10 patients have received their meds and the other 30 patients will have a pass from taking morning medications today. The worst case scenario it that the same nurse could be scheduled to work the next morning, or even worse, the same nurse could be working a double shift the next day.

On this particular day, one of my favorite nurses to work with and I had challenged each other to race passing meds. Both of us being the regular nurses on the unit meant that neither of us held a competitive edge on beating the other, so off we went. Who actually won the challenge on that day, I can't remember, but I can vividly remember, in great detail, everything else that occurred on the particular shift. As my colleague and I sat at the nurse's station swapping stories about all the things that had occurred during our med pass challenge that could have potentially slowed us down, we suddenly heard a disturbing sound. It sounded like a screech, a moan, and a cry of distress. We both stood up and immediately proceeded down our assigned units and began making rounds in and out of each patient's room, making sure to look at each of the faces of every single patient, trying desperately to determine whether anyone had a look of distress on their face. As we met back at the nurse's station, we both looked puzzled and had no idea where the sound had come from. Not sure what to do next, we began running over dinner options of how to proceed from here. Just then, we heard it again. Without any hesitation, my colleague and I immediately charged up and down the hallways and made our rounds in and out of the patients' rooms again, this time with sheer determination that we were going to find out exactly where that sound came from. We were determined; nothing was going to stop us now.

As I backtracked through each room, I made sure to be even more diligent and thorough than I was the first time. I knew that the sound wasn't a good thing; I knew that with my many years of experience, a patient was undoubtedly in danger and they needed immediate assistance. I placed intense scrutiny on each part of the patients' rooms, including checking the bathrooms and closets, something I did not do the first time around. As I reached the very last room, I heard the noise again, only this time, the noise was much louder and more verbose. I was certain that I had finally found the source of that terrifying cry for help. I slowly opened the door, gently bracing myself for what I was going to find, and I saw a sight that I'll never forget. I can recall this image as if I had just seen it. A frail ninety-year-old woman was trapped between the toilet and the wall with her head against the floor, resting in a pool of blood that had already began to coagulate. I frantically called for help. I called out for a Code Blue just to be on the safe side. I knew that she was still alive, but I know by yelling for a Code Blue, it would have received the most attention and the most help in record time. As we waited for the paramedics to arrive we carefully lifted her from where she was lodged into a lying position so that we could apply a pressure dressing to the zigzag-shaped laceration in the middle of her forehead. In the midst of wrapping the bandage, I couldn't help but notice that her laceration was almost identical to that of Frankenstein. Maybe I was trying to find a little humor in a terrible situation, or maybe my emotions were so uncontrolled that humor was the only place that my mind would allow me to go.

As the fire department and paramedics placed the frail woman on the stretcher with the oxygen mask and neck immobilizer, I still managed to see the look of fear in her eyes. She looked terrified. As she was rolled into the elevator, I could hear my director of nursing yelling at me from down the hall.

"How did this happen?" she screamed. "Who was the person that left her at the toilet?!" Those were all good questions, but unfortunately, I did not have answers to her pressing questions. "I want answers!" she demanded.

Now, before you hear my response, I must first explain something about my director of nursing (DON). At this time, the DON was a true commander in chief. She was very straightforward, almost to the point where she could (and often would) instill fear into you just by giving you the look. She always made me a little nervous, and I always tried to do my very best work when I knew she was going to be around for my shift. She ran a very tight ship, and did not play games. If anything was wrong on any nurse's unit, she came down hard on the nurses. She truly ruled with an iron fist. "A unit is a reflection of the nurse that works it," she used to say. I still hear that phrase in my head; when she asked questions, not knowing the answer was never, ever acceptable. Because of her intense and aggressive style of management, I began to fear what was going to happen next. The combination of fear and suspense led me to feel very irate.

Since I was not exactly sure how to handle the situation, I began doing the most simple thing I could think of at the time—I began asking the nursing assistants who had left the patient at the toilet.

Unsurprisingly, no one answered. The room was quiet. You could almost hear the sounds of crickets in the room because of the overwhelming silence after my question. Finally, a CNA stepped up and in a very soft and embarrassed voice embarrassed voice saying, " I did." I felt my head turn in slow motion, trying to locate where the words came from. When I finally acknowledged the individual that was responsible, I became ten times more irate than I was before. This person was the most humble, the most respected, and the very best CNA I have ever met. She was honestly one of the best CNAs on the planet, but none of that mattered right now.

I quickly grabbed the telephone commanding and demanding that, "*You*, the person responsible, come here, come and call the family and tell them that you put their mother, a frail ninety-year-old woman who cannot talk, nor walk, who cannot sit in a regular chair and cannot even feed herself on a toilet and left her all alone!" I screamed.

"Tell her that you left her mom on the toilet and that she fell forward, cracked her forehead on the wall in front of her just as she fell, and got stuck between the toilet and the wall and that we found her upside down with her heading swimming in a cold pool of her own blood!"

I motioned for the CNA to grab the phone. I yelled louder and louder, each time becoming more voracious with my commanding. "You call the family, damn it! Because I'm not! You tell the daughter you left her mother on the toilet to go hang up clothes elsewhere."

There was still no movement. Everyone assigned to the unit stood there at the desk, relieved they weren't the one responsible. Finally, the DON (nickname for director of nursing reappeared and yelled, "ENOUGH! Stop this now!" Still maintaining eye contact, I started to feel bad for what I had just put this CNA through. The D.O.N. then stated that she would make the call to the family and tell them what just happened.

As the team of nursing assistants and nosey ancillary staff dismissed themselves, I couldn't help but notice everyone's disappointment in the way I had spoken to the elder CNA. The truth is that I was correct in saying that you can't leave a person who is total care unattended on the toilet, but I was so wrong, very wrong, when I accused the CNA of being unconcerned and uncaring about her job. The truth is that she was a terrific, loving, caring, and loyal CNA, and it was wrong of me to speak negatively about her because of this one mistake. Although it was a very large mistake that could have had enormous consequences, the patient was still alive. I actually began to feel as sorry for the CNA—almost as much I did for my patient who had fallen. In my entire tenure as a nurse, I have never met a more loyal, compassionate person that genuinely loved every patient.

Never have I met someone that treated each female patient like a sister or mother and each male patient like a brother or father. But why did I feel so bad for reprimanding someone that was so very wrong and negligent? Who was wrong, the CNA or myself? If the CNA walked away from this job right now, who would miss them the most—the patients, that's who! The ones who can't talk but can tell this CNA what their aches and pains are with a simple look in their eyes. Who else would miss the CNA? The patients who have no family to buy them clothes and shoes but are happy that this CNA would never allow them to be without. Who would miss this CNA? The patients who look forward to the small talk and updates on world news while they're being fed, showered, put in bed, or even being put on the toilet every twenty minutes so they don't soil their clothes. Finally, you ask, who would miss this particular CNA? Every nurse who appreciates having eyes and ears and genuine concern day in and day out. No matter how many nurses, CNAs, DONs, as well as administrators come and go, this CNA remains loyal; not to the company but to the patients.

After more than thirty years, how do you not allow for one

mistake? The truth is that people are only human, and humans do make mistakes. The main difference lies in the fact that there is less room to make mistakes when you're a nurse because the stakes are much higher when you're dealing with someone's life! Most occupations do not require the stress and quick thinking that being a nurse does. That responsibility is wonderful to have, but it certainly does create added tension and stress to being a nurse.

The patient returned to the hospital almost a week later. As I entered her room just to see how she was doing, I noticed her smiling. It was almost as if she were expecting me. It was almost as if she was expecting me. The smile on her face, however, wasn't for me. Just as I looked into her eyes, she turned toward the nice CNA that was feeding her and opened her mouth for the next spoonful of oatmeal. Who would miss this CNA? The forgiving patient with the Frankenstein shaped laceration down her forehead. I never said the CNA wasn't wrong for leaving the patient unattended, I'm simply saying that we all make mistakes, sometimes BIG mistakes, but when you are quick to terminate as an immediate plan of correction, you don't just terminate the staff member's employment, you terminate everything that this person has brought and given to the residents. You terminate loving relationships, trusting bonds, and even worse for some of them, the only family they have. What's my point? The next time we're in a position to terminate someone based on how their action on any given day may have impacted our day, maybe we should compare it to how many lives they've impacted everyday, for, let's say, the last thirty years and counting. The bond between a caring, loving CNA and their patient is deep, and it is something that should never, ever be broken or terminated.

In God We Trust

It wasn't until my tenth year of nursing that I realized that I needed God more than ever in my life. By this time, I had worked at three different facilities (unnamed, of course) that had covertly learned to master the art of concealing medical malpractices, medication errors, and other incidents that could have been easily been avoided. Although I cannot say with 100 percent certainty that any of these events ever resulted in a patient's death or permanent damage, I will say, however, that there have been countless times that I have sat in my truck alone and afraid, not sure what was going to happen as a result of these nursing disasters. Plagued with confusing thoughts, I didn't know if I should report these kinds of incidents or not. With tears gently streaming down my face, I prayed to GOD and cried out for HIM to save me and to guide me in the right direction. Order my steps, dear GOD. Although I was never the nurse who was directly involved in any of these unfortunate events, I couldn't help but feel just as guilty knowing the cold hard truth that was being swept under the rug. I couldn't help but think of what would happen if the family only knew the truth. I believe in honesty, dignity, and doing what is right, and I firmly believe that the patients and their loved ones have the right to know the truth, even if it makes a hospital, clinic, or nursing home appear negligent, especially when, in fact, they really are.

There have been many, many times where I've overheard the hospital administrators or the director of nursing feed the families a line of sheer and utter bullshit at its finest. The staff had an infamous reputation for covering up potentially dangerous medication errors, hiding suspected abuse reports, and forcing nurses to edit their nurses' notes so that everything is charted as it should have happened rather than what actually happened. Each time I heard any of the staff members lying to the patients' families, I became physically and emotionally ill. I absolutely love being a nurse, and I wouldn't trade my career choice for the world. I'm hoping that after this book is published, I can still work as a nurse. But the truth is I simply cannot bear the thought of lying to a patient's family and trying to keep the truth from being uncovered. I can't help it. I was born with a strong conscience, and knowing what was going on under the radar at the hospital was beginning to have a profound and understandably negative impact on my physical and mental well-being.

There was one specific incident that still haunts my memory to this very day. This particular incident broke my heart, and it is still difficult for me to write about this event, though it happened many years ago. When this incident occurred, I began praying harder than I have ever prayed in my entire life. I was on my knees begging God from the bottom of my heart to forgive me. I was not asking for forgiveness for anything that I, personally, had done wrong, but for not exposing the truth about those who did wrong. I was asking for forgiveness for not being brave enough to stand up to those who were doing wrong and expose the truth for what it really was. I feel as if it was my Christian duty to do the right thing at all times. Haunted by the guilt of my actions, I can recall going to my granny's house and telling her that I felt that God was disappointed in me because I had selfishly sat there and watched a reputable facility cover up a huge, fatal mess. There is no doubt that this was potentially a huge lawsuit, one that could have gone down in the record books. The implications were sky high for all of the parties involved. My granny responded in the same loving and gentle voice that she always did and said, "Kerrin, after you pray about it, let it go. Put your problems in God's hands." She continued to go on and on in a sermon-like lecture and said, "Strange things start to happen when you start costing people, with a lot of money, a lot of money and their reputation. What's done is done. It was not you who did it and you can't undo it." I don't know whether she scared the hell out of me or if I really just let it go and let God remove the heavy weight of the guilt from my shoulders, but the mere thought of revealing this secret never crossed my mind again until now. My faith tells me that the Lord forgave me, and he knew that I had suffered enough from the guilt of not bringing this issue into light.

I arrived at work an hour early one day. I liked to show up at odd hours to catch the nursing staff off guard to make sure my team is following all of the hospital's policies and procedures when I am not there; however, I also like to make sure that the staffing needs are taken care of and everything is running as smoothly and as efficiently as possible. On this particular day, I stepped out of my flashy Ford Mustang (license plate LPN KJ) only to have a CNA approach me as I closed my door. "He didn't have to die!" she said. Unaware of who this woman was and what she was referring to I gave the woman a puzzled look and shouted, "Huh? Who the hell are you and what the hell are you talking about?" As the woman stood there frantically, she began crumbling on the inside, trying desperately to find the words to say. She was bawling, and then she slowly began explaining the chain of events.

"The guy had his call light on, but he ALWAYS has his call light on, so, we ignored it. I admit we sat at the nurses' station just talking about different things, to be honest. KJ, you know yourself, after a call light has been buzzing for so long, after a while you tend to not even hear it anymore." This was a sad, but very real truth, and I had no choice but to silently nod my head in agreement. "When I finally entered his room, he was holding his neck as if he were choking. Immediately, I ran and called the nurse." For legal purposes, I will refer to this nurse as "Nurse Lorraine". The CNA continued her story: " '201, room 201,' I yelled out. By that time, Nurse Lorraine, the other nurse, and three CNAs had arrived at the room. At this point, the patient had hypersecretion and had rapidly begun turning colors in front of our very eyes. We all stood there, frozen and terrified, desperately regretting the fact that we had all stood there chatting while ignoring his call light for so long. Nobody moved; we just stared. Finally, Nurse Lorraine said, 'Page respiratory, STAT.' Within a minute, the respiratory team had arrived on the scene. As soon as the therapist arrived she yelled for the crash cart and suction machine that had remained behind the nurses' station, untouched throughout all the chaos. The therapist began suctioning the man, but by then he was rapidly turning dark and had stopped moving. There was no pulse, no blood pressure. It was official—he was gone. Nurse Lorraine frantically yelled, 'What's his code status?' The other nurse in the room yelled back, 'DNR!' " The CNA went on to say, "But KJ, they still did CPR for a few minutes, and then they just stopped!" I listened to the CNA tell her story as I created my own visual, slowly replaying every scene in my head. I actually felt as if I were there. Not knowing how to handle the situation, I then urged her not to discuss this with her colleagues, but only to discuss this with her management. I walked in the building as if I knew nothing. I went straight to the second floor, where I saw a staff of nurses and CNAs working as if nothing had just happened. At this point, I did not know what to think. Puzzled by the calm vibe of the floor, I proceeded to reach for the patient's chart. As I found the most recently dated progress notes, they read as follows: "Pt observed during routine rounds unresponsive, not breathing, no blood pressure, and unpalpable pulse," signed Nurse Lorraine. When I questioned Nurse Lorraine about the patient who had just died she simply restated what she had written. She then went on to say that even though he was a DNR, (do not resuscitate) they had still done CPR. I looked at her in utter disbelief. I was amazed that this woman who literally quotes the Bible at every chance she can get would stand here and recite this well-rehearsed lie as if it were the truth. My response to her statement was, "If he was a DNR, why would you do CPR?" I could tell I had caught her off guard. She was not expecting me to question what she had said. Stumbling to come up with a clever response, she then replied, "Well . . . for the sake of doing something." Instantly, I replied by saying, "You say that as if it were questioned that you did nothing." Most of my colleagues expect my quick, comebacks, my dry sarcasm, and of course, my ridiculously smart-ass mouth. But alas, that's just me, that's just KJ. That's what comes to mind when you put those two letters together—smart-mouthed KJ.

By the end of my shift at 3:30 p.m., I was summoned to the administrator's office regarding my report of what had happened, based on the statements that I had taken from the staff on duty when the patient passed away.

First and foremost, the administrator informed me that Nurse Lorraine subsequently changed her statement to say that she didn't initiate CPR, but instead did abdominal thrusts after observing the patient choking during routine rounds. In utter disbelief, my jaw dropped to the floor. He then stated that from that point on he would complete the investigation and instructed me that there would be no further questioning needed by me. Finally, he handed me a form to sign that read:

"I, Kerrin Jackson, was not authorized to discuss any events that may have led up to the death of John Doe. I, unknowingly, submitted false information from several staff members that may be deemed questionable, unethical, and negligible. Any further questioning, verbal, or written submission could result in termination or legal action."

Against my better judgment, I reluctantly placed the pen on the paper and slowly signed the form, questioning myself with each pen stroke. Part of me felt like I was signing my death sentence as I was doing it. In retrospect, I had no choice but to sign the form. After all, I needed my job, and there would be severe repercussions if I had refused to acknowledge and sign the form. I also need to avoid being blackballed as a result of refusing the sign the form. A large part of me felt like, as I signed my name, God was making notes in the Lamb's Book of Life. I hope and pray such notes were a reflection of my good heart and good intent to do the right thing and not of my action that signed and commitment to comply. I concluded that meeting as I conclude this chapter . . . in prayer.

"Our father, who art in Heaven, hallowed be thy name. Thy kingdom come, thy will be done, on earth as it is in Heaven. Give us this day, our daily bread and forgive us our trespasses as we forgive those who trespass against us. Lead us not into temptation, but deliver us from evil, for thine is the kingdom and the power and the glory, forever. Amen."

A Lesson to Learn

Although I'm not the type of person who likes to brag, I have to admit that it was kind of nice that everyone in my family and all of my friends who weren't involved in the medical profession admired me. A lot of them that were, in fact, nurses still valued my opinion and respected my profession, which further validated my career as a nurse. Many times, my family and friends (and friends of my family and family of my friends' family as well) would constantly look to me for "the truth" when it came to interpreting and translating what their doctors were trying to avoid telling them. Sometimes, they just couldn't get a straight answer from their doctors, and that's where I would step in.

The truth is, I did enjoy showing off my nursing skills, whether it was to family, patients, patients' families, or coworkers. This included doctors as well. There have been a few times where people would ask me to act as a liaison between them and the physician. Usually, if I started conversing with the physician directly, it didn't take them long to realize I was in the medical profession, which prompted the infamous question from the doctor, "Are you a nurse? " I anticipated this question. I couldn't wait for this question. I always had the same reply, "With all due respect, Doctor, this discussion is about your patient, not me." They would eventually figure it out. None, however, had any idea that I was an LPN, not an RN. After their question, my response usually prompted a stern look followed by a detailed briefing of what was actually going on with the patient. After the mini power struggle, I would explain to the family in layman's terms (non-clinical terminology) so that they could understand exactly what I was saying, rather than speaking in medical terminology as most doctors and nurses have a tendency to do.

Sometimes I can't help but wonder if those doctors and nurses are secretly hoping that families will feel too dumb to ask questions or keep asking the doctor repeatedly to explain when they simply don't understand something they've said. This is all too common, and the harsh reality is that this tends to work most of the time!

After you've spent hours in the emergency room, hoping and praying that God will fix this and make you better again, the doctor comes in to explain what the problem is, and as soon as he leaves, you are left clueless about what he just said because he spoke in medical terminology the entire time and he spoke to the patients in the same language as if he were speaking to another doctor or nurse, which is not the way that patients need to be spoken to! The patient doesn't understand what is wrong with them or how they can fix their ailment.

A perfect example of what I am saying: once I heard a doctor tell a patient's family member, "Your mother is lethargic due to her low hemoglobin. Also, her urinary output is minimal, so we'll get a basic metabolic profile, BUN, and creatine, check her electrolytes, and do a CT of her brain just to make sure she didn't have a CVA. But in the meantime we'll get some fluids in her."

Unless you're a seasoned professional in the medical field you probably have no idea what I'm talking about, just as most family members wouldn't know, and you shouldn't have to, either. After all, the average layperson isn't trained to know these things; that is what doctors and nurses are for. I recall a moment in my nursing career when I was actually on the "other side" of the nurse's station, and let me tell you, it is not the easiest thing in the world to do. I had learned from my mother, in May of 2008, that my godmother (Sweet Mary, I called her) had actually been to a scheduled doctor's appointment and ended up hospitalized. The next day, I learned that she wasn't doing well, so I immediately hopped in the car and sped to the hospital on 1st Avenue to check on her. When I arrived, she was unresponsive and hooked up to a ventilator. Her vital signs were 72/40, 57, 16, 97.9. She didn't look good, and it didn't take a nursing degree to see that she was not doing well. I was devastated. With tears running down my face, I asked the nurse what had happened. Unfortunately, the nurse wasn't helpful at all. She said, "She drove herself over for a routine appointment, and now she is on a ventilator." In young person terminology, I could help but think, "WTF?" Not sure what to say next, she responded by saying, "I'm not sure; I haven't seen the emergency room's notes, but I can get the doctor who can tell you more." I agreed to speak with the doctor as I wiped a handful of tears on my sleeve.

About fifteen minutes later, a tall, thin man walked into the room. He was wearing a doctor's lab coat with an expensive stethoscope around his neck. He extended his arm for a handshake as he introduced himself. "Hi, I'm Michael Anthony. I am taking care of your godmother, Mary. The nurse said you had some questions for me." Not wanting to waste any more time beating around the bush, I asked the doctor to brief me on what was going on. The conversation went as follows:

Doctor: "Well, right now her BP is low so we are giving her 12 mcg of Levophed. We're also giving her 0.2mg of Neo-Synephrine through her IV. We think she may be septic. We're going to start her on some broad-spectrum antibiotics until we get back some of her cultures. The nurse is going to get some urine from her shortly, and hopefully by this afternoon we'll have an idea of what kind of antibiotic to give her based on her sensitivity and resistant report. Also, we placed her on a mechanical ventilation apparatus, because in the past she had an episode of respiratory arrest where she desaturated, so just prophylactically we put her on a vent in case she should arrest."

I could tell by the preserved half grin he was hiding he felt like he had just triumphed. Indeed, he sounded like a great doctor; however, he wasn't a doctor, and that was solely the problem.

Me: "Hello, Mr. Anthony. There must be a mistake. I asked to speak with a doctor. You are clearly a resident, not a physician, which is why you introduced yourself by your full name. Every decision that you make has to be approved by your senior. Basically, all you've told me is that you suspect she has a very bad infection. You're not sure if it's in her blood, or urine. You're not even sure that it's an infection, but for insurance purposes, let call it "sepsis." Then you tell me you're going to culture both blood and urine in the morning, and get results back a few hours later, then put her on an antibiotic most sensitive based on the report. Excuse me, sir . . . a urinalysis, yes, a CBC, WBC, BUN, creatine, yes, yes, yes. Culture and sensitivity results in a couple hours? NO, NO, and NO. It takes days for a culture to grow; don't insult my intelligence! Then, you are telling me that you put her on a ventilator even though she did not go into respiratory arrest, nor did she desaturate. You put her on a got damn ventilator for no apparent reason, and now she lays comatose and nobody has any idea as to why! Is that why they sent the third year resident doctor-in-training to tell me?"

At this point, I'm screaming and wiping tears in front of this kid-looking student who hasn't even learned not to get emotional about patients, which is one of the first things you need to know before getting involved in the medical field! Staring directly into his eyes, I thought he was going to cry, too. In the back of my mind, I knew that no matter how ignorant I became and made a spectacle of myself it didn't change her condition. And being a nurse of seventeen years, I knew her condition wasn't going to change either . . . at least not for the better. My sweet, kind, loving godmother passed away two days later, after driving herself to a routine doctor's appointment. What happened? Who knows? At a teaching hospital, it's not important whether the patient lives or dies—what's important is that the students learn from their mistakes . . . and a mistake was definitely made. The question is not what was the cause of her dying, but more importantly, did she die for a good cause?

Politics in Nursing

It wasn't until I was promoted to a unit coordinator that I realized that politics play a substantial role in nursing. It seemed as if the patients came second, and money came first, which is something I really didn't understand. The motto around the hospital quickly became, "If it doesn't make dollars, it doesn't make sense." It was then that I suddenly learned that the primary objective of the administrators and owners was to simply spend as little as they possibly could so they could end up saving more money—go figure! This notion was explained in detail to me by a former assistant director of nursing. She claimed that the hospital's owners would offer her a $25,000 bonus if she managed to keep the facility under the allocated annual budget each fiscal year. Because the bonus incentive was quite lucrative, the administrator would do anything they could to make sure that they never even came close to overrunning the budget and potentially losing their end-of-the-year bonus. The administrator would call a department meeting and sell the employees on the idea that each department was already overspending and that they were already WAY over their annual budget, and therefore, jobs may need to be cut as a result. Obviously, at this point, the staff members of each department were terrified of losing their jobs and being unemployed. Because of their fear and strong emotional desire to keep their jobs, they were willing to do nearly anything to remain employed.

This is the time when the administrator would sneakily "propose a solution": "

If, and only *if,* each of you (including the dietary supervisor, housekeeping supervisor, director of nursing, activity director, rehab director, and maintenance director) can strategically cut some costs from their budget starting immediately, there is a strong possibility that we can save everyone's job." If that isn't enough motivation, the administrator also agrees to offer them an additional $5,000 bonus each if they stay under the allowed budget by January. At this point, every supervisor in the building is now on the same page. This is how the scenario takes shape, and subsequently, budgets are drastically cut. There are more sandwiches served instead of actual dinners, from pieces of chicken to chicken nuggets; from pure apple/orange juice to fruit drink; from durable laundry bags to paper thin plastic that tear in an instant; from Dial soup to a generic green body wash that is shampoo and conditioner all in one—gross! And hand lotion . . . that is also included in the body wash, if you can believe it!

In nursing, house stock could typically be found everywhere EXCEPT in the house itself, of course. Let me clarify that statement. House stock can be found everywhere except the facility. It's not uncommon, however to visit a coworker and find everything I'm looking for at their house—but that's another chapter. Enteric coast aspirin, ferrous sulfate, calcium supplements, and even Colace were considered hot commodities. I used to joke that the nurses were like squirrels, hiding supplies so they would have them ready for their shift as soon as we ran out. As if this wasn't bad enough, it didn't stop there . . . not even close. Alcohol wipes were literally torn in half for double use. One side of the wipe was used to perform an Accu-Check, while the other side was strategically used to administer the insulin injection that usually went along with it. There's a good chance that my career may be blackballed in the nursing world after this book lands on the right desk—or shall I say the "wrong desk"—so I may as well confess everything now and be an open book—pun intended.

Over the course of my career, I have worked at several facilities were there was a severe shortage of Accu-Check strips or insulin syringes, and I, myself as well as others, have been forced to choose which patients to use the last supplies for, which is very morally and ethically wrong; however, as pretentious as it may sound, this is exactly what we did. After all, what choice did we have? There were so many times this happened and I felt sick to my stomach each time. I knew it was wrong, and just because they are cutting budgets doesn't mean that the patients should have to suffer as a result. That is morally wrong, and playing favoritism on which patients receive the last of the supplies is cruel and unusual, and it also leads to other legal and ethical issues like discrimination.

Patients who had chronic normal blood sugar were always bypassed so that we could use the supplies for those who were unstable with their diabetes or labeled as "brittle diabetics," as we referred to them as. It didn't matter how many times you ordered supplies from the stock person, or how many times you'd go to the stock room yourself, there were NEVER any supplies!

Once it had been officially determined that we had successfully managed to slide underneath the annual budget and a new fiscal year began, things would go back to normal— temporarily, that is. As soon as the fiscal year came close to culminating, the same vicious cycle would rear its ugly head once again and then everyone would begin hiding supplies and selfishly deciding which patients would receive which supplies. On the nursing units, we just appreciated having the supplies we needed so that we could go home and actually enjoy the families we seldom saw, instead of worrying, wondering, and praying that one person who didn't get this Accu-Check done didn't end up in a diabetic coma in his sleep because the one day we skipped over him he actually needed his insulin to survive.

Did I ever mention how many times CNAs couldn't do their rounds because there were no linens or towels? Also, how the residents didn't get their clothes back from laundry in a timely manner due to the skeleton crew that each department had staffed? Unlike Washington politics, you don't get to vote on the changes being implemented or the programs being cut. Nope! You are forced to roll with the punches and deal with it. You wouldn't even dare have the audacity to approach upper-level management, either, as they are only concerned about the money, not the patient's health, safety, or overall experience in our hospital. Neither do you get the vote for the people in offices that are making those changes. While there may not be any Democrats versus Republicans in the medical field, politics are quite prevalent in the nursing field—far more than people typically think. While hospital administration and owners resemble kings and queens riding atop elephants in royal fashion, we, the other political party, stand there like asses, hoping and waiting for a wave, a hello, or to be called on by name as the parade takes place. Elephants and asses, that's definitely politics in the nursing world! As unfortunate as it may sound, it is the truth, for all that it really is underneath the false charade—or shall I say false parade?

My Crew

Right from the beginning of day one, it was quite evident that not everyone on my team was a team player—even those employees that exemplified the natural talents and abilities to perform as team players had their bad days. My immediate supervisor, the ADON (assistant director of nursing), was a no-nonsense, "super" supervisor nurse that never had a "laid back" day at work. She was tough, and many of the other employees feared her as she commanded orders and demands from her staff. Each and every day, she laid down the law and we did our very best to be law-abiding citizens. We could almost sense the way the vibe in the room changed when her little red Ford Festiva pulled into the parking lot. A grim feeling came over me, and I always knew she was on her way in. It was the very thought of her that everything—and I do mean everything—had to be perfect. If anything fell short of sheer perfection, I was the first person that she summoned to her office to get reprimanded. I never admitted it before now, but even I was fearful of her. She had this cutting edge in the manner in which she spoke that made everything she had to say seem as if razors were attached. I strived for perfection when I worked under her supervision.

She was very, very keen on appearance—appearance of the unit, and appearance of the patients, too. It didn't matter what was going on in any of our personal lives, and it didn't matter how slammed we were taking care of other patients. She made it crystal clear that all patient's beds had to be made before 10 a.m.; otherwise, all hell would break loose, and none of us wanted to be there to face the wrath of her rage. None of us ever wanted to push her buttons or test her on her word, so we eagerly obliged to her demands, no matter how outrageous some of them seemed. Most of us would inherently make sure their assignment was near perfect long before the 10 a.m. deadline; however, nurses are only human, and every now and then there was one of us that would be having a bad day. An example of a typical day is as follows:

It's 9:30am and the most difficult part of the chaotic morning rush has finally come to an end. The nursing staff feels accomplished and proud of their work. All of the patients are out of bed, bathed, and fed. Rather than rejoicing in our work, someone checks their watch and it says 9:35 a.m. Suddenly, one of the nurses runs to the window only to feel their stomach churn and an emotional wave of fear come over them as they witness a small red Festivia slowly pulling into the parking lot.

When the nurses see this, the "code" is anxiously announced throughout the entire unit in an attempt to give everyone a "heads up" that the otherwise peaceful morning is coming to a screeching halt. At that time, everybody frantically begins making their last rounds to ensure that their unit is absolutely perfect; otherwise, they know what is in store for them when the boss arrives. At that very moment, I realize that one of the CNAs still has two patients in bed and six beds that have not yet been made. I am quite frightened as to what I am witnessing. Without hesitation, I immediately announce for all four CNAs to quickly come to the nurse's station. After all of the CNAs arrive at the nurse's station, I say, "There are six beds that still need to be made ASAP in the third group. We have five minutes to make it happen. We can do it! Come on, team! Let's go!" These are dreaded words, and nobody likes to comply. After all, why should they? Nobody likes to do someone else's work. The extent to how angry the CNAs would become when asked to perform someone else's task would depend on why, in fact, the CNA didn't finish her own work. The usual excuses varied from them not feeling well, to which they weren't too upset. If they were nursing a hangover, though, the others were mildly upset. If the CNA was goofing off all morning and wasting time, they were undoubtedly pissed off.

Nevertheless, when the storm came, the nurses all stuck together and acted like a unified team to get the work finished in a timely manner. I used to always close my announcement with, "Don't get upset. It might be *you* who is having a bad day tomorrow." The nurses understood. By the time lunchtime rolled around, everybody was OK, and there was nothing new. This was a typical day, and not any different from any other day. The nurses argued, they disagreed, and although we worked together, we still liked to get together and socialize outside of work. We borrowed money from each other, hitched rides, we bought each other lunch, we shared secrets, we told secrets, we even told secrets we weren't supposed to tell. The bottom line is, we were family and those are the things that family does. It's almost impossible not to be like family with your fellow nurses, since you do so much together and you spend so much time together. You learn from each other, you bond with each other, and you grow together.

Interestingly enough, not all of my nursing memoirs are nightmares; there are many happy, fulfilling moments that are part of my career that I wouldn't trade for the world. I truly love being a nurse. I had not one, but two separate opportunities to work with an all-star crew on the fourth floor of my favorite job. This wasn't an ordinary team of CNA's; it was a team of housekeepers, activity aides, and restorative aides, not to mention the other nurse who worked beside me, my "P" (for partner) is what she called me. We all complimented each other in every aspect of the word. We were far more than colleagues. We were family, and family is among the strongest of bonds that exist. We mentored each other. We supported each other. We encouraged each other, and we all cared deeply for each other as people. This was my definition of "The Dream Team."

Each and every floor in the building envied the fourth floor, for obvious reasons. Of course, we couldn't help but brag a little. Since we ran our unit perfectly, like a well-oiled machine or an efficient assembly line at a manufacturing plant, we earned our bragging rights for those reasons. The only difference between an assembly line's productivity and ours is that we didn't use robotics; we used our hearts. We had real, genuine relationships with our patients, which is something that you cannot learn in nursing school or medical school. Bedside manner is a skill that, quite frankly, cannot be taught. Some doctors and nurses have it, and others do not—it's that simple. We brought our patients clothes and shoes from our own homes. We brought them small, quality lotions and hair accessories, and all of the small, minute things they needed. They were more than just patients to us. They were our family, and you take care of your family at all costs. Doing small, kind gestures for our patients was how we showed them that we cared about them, and unfortunately, that kind of treatment is uncommon in most hospitals today. Once, during a public health survey, one of the surveyors found our floor and was amazed at what she witnessed. During the exit interview (when public health was finished investigating), the surveyor included the following in her report:

"Never in my thirty-year career have I seen a dementia unit so organized, and run so well. The relationship between the staff is the epitome of what teamwork truly is. I am quite impressed!"

While receiving a compliment on your performance always gives you that warm, snug feeling inside, receiving a compliment like that from the state only comes once in a lifetime. It felt incredible to receive that type of compliment, and hearing it once reinforced my beliefs as what teamwork truly is, and how lucky I was to manage such an excellent team. Again, I had the wonderful opportunity of hearing it twice, same unit, just a different cast and crew—*my crew.*

911 to 119

Many times, newspapers, television, and word of mouth have a strange way of shining a dismal and gruesome light on nursing home care, as well as the nurses and CNAs that work in them. Although the media has the power to perpetually label nursing home care this way, a vast majority of the time we nurses do the best we can with what we have to work with, which isn't much most of the time. The general public doesn't realize that most of the time we are working with extremely limited resources. From having only a small fraction of the supplies we need, doctors not calling us back for hours and hours, and working short-staffed nearly all the time, we are doing pretty well given the circumstances.

When the average layperson compares hospital nursing care to nursing home care, the nursing home nurses always seem to finish last. These results beg the obvious question—are hospital nurses clinically smarter or more knowledgably? Sadly enough, the answer to that loaded question depends on whom you ask; however, on December 20, 2006, my answer would have clearly been based on the following information.

I remember this particular day perfectly. If there was such a thing as "bad luck," I saw it on December 20th. At the nursing home I was working at, we were expecting several new patients to be transferred from various hospitals in the city. On a good day, an experienced nurse from the hospital would call the nursing home and give that nurse a report on the patient to be transferred. A report typically includes a list of diagnoses, the patient's medical history, most recent vital signs, as well as other important medical procedures that were performed during their hospital stay. On this particular day, however, nothing had gone according to standard policy and procedure. No nursing report had been called in when the Stat Ambulance Company rolled a patient through the front door of Valley Rehab and Retirement Center. Since we were expecting the patent, we directed the drivers to room 119. The nurse on the floor was brand new, fresh out of school, and was of course baffled because it initially looked as if the patient was dead. As we slowly walked in the patient's room to put the patient on oxygen, the ambulance driver stated his heart was only functioning at 20 percent. With a sarcastic tone and demeanor, he shouted, "Good luck!"

Terrified by what I was witnessing literally right before eyes, I froze for a brief moment, but then quickly regained control of my racing, pessimistic thoughts. As the supervisor in charge, I immediately instructed the nurse to page the physician and send the patient back to the hospital ASAP. To my complete and utter surprise, the physician called back in a matter of two minutes. With the report he had received from the rookie nurse, and listening to the sound of fear resonating within her body, he gave the audacious order to send the patient out immediately. A colossal sign of relief from the nurse was heard from two rooms away. It took the paramedics about four minutes to arrive, although it felt like much longer given our anticipation and anxiousness. I motioned for the rookie nurse to escort the paramedics to room 119 so she would be able to chart what the paramedics said while still in the building. Besides, I can recall one specific incident when an ambulance driver came to pick up a patient, and while they were transferring the patient from the bed to the stretcher, they dropped the patient! And if that wasn't bad enough, they tried to hide it from the nursing home! They simply lifted him up from the ground, transported him to the hospital, and pretended nothing had happened. They acted like their job was done. It was during the emergency room assessment that it was determined that the patient had a broken hip as the result of the negligent emergency responder team. In the wonderful world of nursing, that spells out r-e-p-o-r-t-a-b-l-e. Gilroy's Hospital reported this particular nursing home to the state of Illinois and by the following Monday morning, public health was all over the place. In the end, the results were ugly. The nursing home was fined heavily, received a tag, and the family filed a huge law suit for negligence. Two years later, during the court proceedings for this case, it was revealed that the patient had been dropped by the ambulance drivers. Since that time, I make sure to watch them from the time they arrive until the time they leave the building. Nobody is going to drop a patient and try to cover it up on my watch!

Nonetheless, when the paramedics entered room 119 at Valley Nursing Home, they observed a man looking almost lifeless. His vital signs were not much different than from when the nurse took them. As the paramedics slowly rolled the patient from room 119 down the hall toward the front door, we heard one of them boldly shout, "Code Blue Now! Code Blue Now!" At that very moment, right in the center of the main lobby, CPR was being performed on the patient. After a few minutes of unsuccessful attempts at CPR, the patient was rolled to the ambulance and driven away.

Although I was nearly certain that he wasn't going to make it, we waited for about twenty minutes before we received a call from the hospital to confirm our worst fears—the man had passed away. Approximately five minutes after that phone call, we received a call from a different nearby hospital informing us that we would be receiving a patient that had previously been at our facility. Although I didn't have a room ready for this patient, and the mere fact that the last twenty minutes had drained me from all my emotional and physical reserve energy, I simply said, "Okay." The first thought that popped into my head was one of relief. I was happy that at least they had called to inform us.

After the chaos had slowly calmed down from the previous admission and the housekeeping crew was finished cleaning room 119, the next admission rolled in. "What room?" the ambulance driver asked. The rookie nurse mumbled in a low, timid voice, "Room 119." The ambulance driver didn't know what to make of her response. Nevertheless, he transported the patient to room 119 as he was instructed to. At 11:30 p.m., things were dead quiet. The p.m. graveyard shift was lingering around discussing and reporting everything that had recently transpired on the 3 p.m. to 11 p.m. shift. Normally, the overhead paging system is off-limits on the nightshift, but what happened next was certainly an exception to the rule. "Code Blue room 119, Code Blue room 119!" Hoping and praying that this was all nothing more than a big misunderstanding, I shouted, "You have got to be kidding me! Please be kidding! Damn it! God, please!" As we carefully initiated a Code Blue and began CPR, the very same 911 crew that had just left came back. They performed CPR on the woman for several minutes before rolling her out of the building and into the ambulance. Just like the person who occupied that room no more than one hour ago, I did not expect this woman to make it either. As grim as that sounds, all of my years of schooling and training told me that she was going to pass away as well, and my medical intuition is usually correct. Determined to have just a single personal moment to myself to regroup my thoughts and emotions, I walked toward my office located on the first floor. I was mesmerized by how good it felt to sit and relax on the big, comfy office chair. My feet were tired, although I was physically exhausted and could not believe the night I had just experienced. Thinking I may be in the midst of a nightmare, I pinched myself to make sure I wasn't away in a deep slumber. I didn't know if I could take anymore of this. As I sat quietly at my desk, I found myself mindlessly doodling on an oversized calendar.

It's almost as if the room was haunted, and it had claimed two lives in one evening, which is quite rare. Strangely enough, I didn't even realize I had been on a roll writing the same number, "119," over and over. I thought about counting how many times I had actually written the number down. With my luck, it probably would have turned out to be 119 times! Closing my eyes and praying that this was the last death this room would ever see, I turned my fears to the Lord and said a prayer. All things are possible through Christ, and hopefully, this was no exception.

And So It Was

When I stop and reminisce about the many variables in my life that led me to the path of becoming a nurse, I cannot help but believe it was a collage of both people and events in my life that inspired and encouraged me to take this path in life. Of course, there are a few in particular that stand out more than others; however, there are many people and events in my life that influenced my career decision. There was my mother, Anna Jackson, who was a retired nurse of over forty years who played the largest role in my decision. I also carry a profound memory of a nurse I knew from many years ago that still haunts me to this very day. Although I don't actually know her, one thing is certainly clear—I have never forgotten her!

My entire life, I can always remember being a sickly child, and even now as a grown adult with a child of my own, I still have not outgrown that particular trait of mine. I can recollect vivid memories of being in what I learned was Cook County Hospital for what seemed like my entire childhood. Back in that day and age, the cribs had an amazing likeness to an animal cage at the zoo, which isn't a surprise considering they were probably made by the same manufacturer. The hospital was dark, cold, and gray. It was a depressing atmosphere and bore a strong odor of Betadine.

As a young child, I had no idea why I was always in this place. The only thing I knew was that everything made me itch all over my body, and I was constantly covered in sores from heavy, continuous scratching to try and ease the pain the only way I knew how. It seemed as if I was always allergic to everything, and even in adulthood, nothing has changed. Every time I came even in the slightest contact with something new that I was allergic to, I would obsessively go on a scratching rampage and before I knew it, I was headed right back to the hospital.

Growing up as a sickly child, I felt a lot of love from my mother, and other members of my family as well. Everybody would come visit me in the hospital and offer comfort and support during these difficult times for me. Their mere presence made me feel warm and safe. I would watch them show up, one by one, and watch them leave in the very same way. The first person to arrive would typically be the first to leave. They would announce that they were leaving. They would say, "I'm looking forward to the candy machine!" The second person who arrived would say, "Well . . . I'm going to check on the first person." This continued on and on until it dwindled down to one single person who would always be standing there with me, my mother, of course. At some point, my mother would usually say to me, "I have to go and check on your sister, Kim."

One early morning, a stone-faced nurse made her way into my room. She didn't make a sound or say a word, yet just her presence made me feel uneasy and scared. She immediately flipped the light on, placed a tiny breakfast tray in front of me, and proceeded to remove me from my "cage." With one hand, she reached into the cage and clipped me with one arm and sat me down at the miniature table area in front of my tray. Next, she untied the cloth diaper that was tightly tied around my hand. It was this cloth diaper that kept me from scratching myself. Although the breakfast cereal placed in front of me resembled Cheerios, it was tasteless and bland, almost like I was eating absolutely nothing at all. It's ironic in a way that I can recall detail after detail of this "breakfast from hell," as I referred to it, yet I can't remember what I had for dinner two days ago!

As I began slowly eating the tasteless cereal, trying to get it down as fast as possible without choking on its flavorless contents, I can vividly recall that I instantly began itching at that very moment. One by one, the hives rapidly began penetrating my skin and popping out of my arms and legs. The feeling was so intense that I had a very hard time sitting still. They itched so badly I wanted to scream at the top of my lungs! I anxiously looked at the barrage of hives forming on top of scratches and bruises that were from the last scratching frenzy. I didn't want to scratch, as I kept thinking of how angry my mother and the nurse would be if I did. I was scared of the nurse, even when I was obeying her commands, and I couldn't even fathom the thought of how angry she would be if I disobeyed her commanding orders.

Still, knowing this, I couldn't help it. Although I tried everything within my power not to scratch, I remember that my left hand just took off scratching, almost as if it had a mind of its own. Every area of skin on my body itched tremendously, and I scratched every area that I could, desperately trying to gain even just a brief moment of temporary relief for my efforts. It felt so good, too! The harder I scratched, the better it felt. Finally, I decided to use my unbandaged hand to unbandage my right hand. Now, I had two hands free, and two hands for scratching are far better than one! Finally, when the itching began to calm, I noticed my arms, hands, legs, and face were covered in blood! It was such a gory, frightening scene for a young child like myself to witness! My scratches were bleeding and my little, ten-year-old face was beet red. My hands and fingernails looked as if I had been finger painting with red paint.

Just as I looked down at my legs, I could see the white nylon leggings that belonged to the nurse who had been in room just moments ago. Slowly, I moved my head upward, and when our eyes met, she was definitely not smiling. In fact, she had a look of sheer anger and disgust on her face. At that time, she began yelling at me, picking up the bloody diaper that was wrapped around my left hand. As I slowly glanced at the neglected, soggy bowl of tasteless cereal, the nurse proceeded to angrily put me right back in my cage and slammed the metal cage door down with great force. It was obvious that she was extremely upset, but I was in a lot of pain, and I couldn't help but to give in and scratch in an effort to relieve my pain. She didn't understand what I was going through, no one did really, and thus, I can recall feeling misunderstood, alone, and in despair.

Although I lay in my cage cold, bloody, and hungry, feeling like a wild animal that had just been captured, I can honestly say that it felt better than itching, oddly enough. Feeling scared, timid, and uneasy about what had just happened, I wanted to tell the nurse I was sorry, but I knew that I would most likely be in the same predicament tomorrow and the next day after that, too. This experience had a profound effect on me, one that would last a lifetime. I never forgot this nurse, nor have I forgotten this traumatic experience. I have replayed this scene hundreds of times in my mind throughout the course of my life. In retrospect, I cannot help but stop and wonder if this nurse ever gained more compassion for her patients. After all, I wondered, why did she become a nurse if she couldn't handle the patients? I wondered if she ever knew how she affected my life, even forty-plus years later. I truly hated her, and I still do, even to this day. Nonetheless, she is the first person who taught me the importance of bedside manner, and how not having proper beside manner could continue to haunt patients for many years and years to come.

The sad reality is that, over the course of my lifetime, I've met so many nurses that reminded me of her, both with nurses that I've worked alongside and nurses that I've had in various hospital stays. Nurses with no heart; nurses with no soul. Some nurses actually go as far as to wear colorful scrubs and act as if they're fun to work with, but they secretly use great force and roughly handle the residents with no regard to their fragile physical and mental state.

Somewhere in a hospital or nursing home, a sick patient is lying very still and very quiet, thinking about that one nurse they were always terrified of, that one nurse who treated them so poorly, just because they needed a simple pain pill at a time most inconvenient for that nurse. A frail, eighty-year-old woman lies in bed, scared to death, because she had another diarrhea episode this shift and she knows the nursing assistant assigned to her will be furious and enraged, and she will suffer the terrible consequences that follow for simply being incontinent. The most that a frail woman could hope for is that the "mean" nursing assistant would at least tell the nurse about the diarrhea so she could get Imodium or Pepto-Bismol to stop it. If not, the next shift CNA will punish her the exact same way. This could go on for days, and sadly, it usually does, and it usually goes under the radar, unnoticed by the management staff at the hospital. For those not offended, be not offended. For those feeling "some kind of way," simply stop "being" that kind of way. Someday, our mothers, fathers, and we ourselves will be that frail patient. Perhaps an addendum to the oath we take could read, "I promise to always be the nurse that I would want for my mother, my grandmother, my child, and myself."

Grapes of Wrath

I can recall this specific event as if I were right there, witnessing it happen right in front of my very eyes. In fact, I was right there, slowly taking in each minute's detail as it happened, second by second.

The crowded restaurant was dead quiet, almost to where I could hear a needle drop to the floor. The people there continued to converse with each other, but I could hear nothing. My ears were popping, sort of like I was on an airplane. My eyes began to fill with tears as I could slowly feel my body begin to panic. Stunned by what was happening to me, I finally realized the inevitable truth of what was happening to me: I was choking!

I had been eating grape after grape after grape until suddenly, my whole world around me just froze, and the symptoms of panic began rearing their ugly head inside of my body. I was terrified, and paralyzed with fear. I can remember frantically thinking, "Why can't anybody in this crowded room see me? Help Me! Somebody!" I screamed as loud as I could, but with the intense choking I was facing, barely a sound came from my throat, and no one turned around at my muffled, bloodcurdling screams.

In a desperate panic to save my life, I started thinking of anything I could do to stop the choking. First, I tried coughing as a method to dislodge the grape. I reached my fingers down my throat to manually remove it myself, but nothing seemed to work. I became so weak and tired very quickly. I realized I was almost out of time, and I had to do something. I couldn't save myself. Someone else had to help me. I needed help now, not two minutes from now—I needed it right then and there. Otherwise, I could very easily wind up dead within another minute or so.

In one motion, using both of my hands, I grabbed the tablecloth tightly and swept everything on our table to the floor. Glasses filled with water, plates with salad went flying, and the table was completely clear within a mere two seconds. The loud, frightening noise of glass being shattered on the hard floor immediately prompted the people in the restaurant to finally turn around to see what was going out. The deafening sound of the dishes cracking on the floor sent shockwaves down the spines of the people eating in the restaurant. Their heads quickly swung around in a frenzy, even in greater dismay when I used my hands to motion that I was rapidly choking.

Suddenly, out of nowhere, a tall middle-aged, well-dressed man in a suit shoved his way through the restaurant, pushing past a crowd of people on their feet. I could see he was mouthing words, but still I could hear nothing. The stranger's face became more and more red as he approached me, and it felt as if my world was in slow motion. He literally tackled me as he flung his arms around my body. I felt a squeeze so strong it could have forced my insides to come up, then another, then another, then another! I could see everyone watching in fear, not knowing what to do next other than to watch this man do his best to save my life.

As the man continued with the Heimlich maneuver, I felt myself regretfully letting go. I was becoming weaker and weaker due to a lack of oxygen. My legs were frail, and felt as if they were going to give out at any moment, leading my body to collapse to the ground. The middle-aged man in the suit must have been in tip-top shape because with both arms already around my waste he picked my limp body up and continued, only this time it was harder and faster than before. As he squeezed me harder with all of his might, I heard an echo, and I heard him say, "Come on . . . come on . . . come on!"

Although his words were faint, I can vividly recall hearing them. The man continued squeezing, and finally I heard him loud and clear as the content that had been lodged in the back of my throat projected out across the room. I started crying out loud with full force. Although I was still frightened and very shaken up by what I had just experienced, I was so relived, and I was elated and so thankful for this man. I wanted to kiss the ground and thank Jesus. This man was truly a blessing to me. It was almost like God had sent this man to be my savior in my darkest hour. The strange man slowly eased me to the floor as the paramedics abruptly arrived on the scene moments later. I can vividly recall staring at the man, and mouthing the words, "Thank you," as the paramedics blocked my view of him.

I spent the next three days in the hospital complaining of cephalalgia (severe headaches). It wasn't until my fourth day in the hospital that it was determined that I was leaking spinal fluid from a spinal tap that caused the severe headaches. Initially, it was speculated that I might have ruptured a small vessel in my brain during the choking episode. A spinal tap was performed and ruled this medical guess incorrect; however, not only does a spinal tap itself cause headaches, but it has the potential to leak fluid, which it most certainly did.

At the end of day four in the hospital, an epidural blood patch was ordered by the doctor. A blood patch is a surgical procedure that uses autologous blood in order to close one or many holes in the dura mater of the spinal cord, usually as a result of a previous lumbar puncture. It was also be used to relieve past dura puncture headaches caused by a lumbar puncture. On day five, I was prepped for the procedure that was to follow. As a gentleman of African descent entered my room, I noticed he was wearing cargo pants, a polo shirt, and a lab jacket. He introduced himself as the physician who would be performing my procedure. Not only was I surprised to learn that the procedure would be done at my bedside, but I was even more surprised to learn that I would be awake during my procedure.

And so the procedure was underway . . .

First, the doctor asked my visitor who had been there beside me to leave the room. "This should only take a half hour," he said. Although it took many attempts to draw my own blood, he was finally ready to infuse my blood into my spinal column to repair the spinal fluid leak. The first injection was lidocaine. As I leaned into a fetal position, I could feel the needle going in as I was bracing myself for the pain that was coming. Next, I saw him pick up the blood-soaked syringe and proceed to inject it into my body.

"Ouch, shit! That fucking hurts!" I screamed! Very surprised by what he had just heard, the doctor looked at me with a puzzled look and said, "You can feel that?" I couldn't help but be a bit sarcastic as I said, "Uhhh . . . yeah!"

"Let me give you more lidocaine, then," he said.

As he finished the second injection of lidocaine, he proceeded to inject the blood before it began to clot in the syringe. I could still feel the larger, more robust needle penetrating my skin, but this time I said nothing. I just wanted him to get it over with as quickly as possible. As the blood pushed through the syringe, I could feel a sudden, alarmingly warm sensation spreading across my back. Naturally, I became scared. I remember screaming, "Something is wrong—I can feel it! It's in my back! It's in my shoulder! It's in my left arm—it's coming back up my arm!" then I blacked out. The next memory I have is waking up to a room packed with nurses and doctors and a crash cart. I had no clue what was going on. I didn't even know why I was there in the hospital to begin with.

I looked around and spotted my former director of nursing, who was now a nurse manager at this hospital. I saw my primary care physician there at the foot of my bed, demanding answers and giving orders to the other doctors and nurses in the room. I saw a man in cargo pants and a polo shirt in the doorway staring at me. I stared back, thinking "Who is he?" The stare was immediately broken when I heard my doctor, Dr. Vaughn, yelling at everyone, "Blood pressure, now!" The nurse said I had a 69/52, 92 pulse. I stared at my doctor in awe, as I always loved to watch him in action. I worked with him for years, watching him be the awesome doctor he is, until I convinced every person in our family to make him their primary care physician as well.

"Give her .9 normal saline, full strength, let's get a CBC ASAP." He made his way to me, calmly explaining everything that was going on. "Kerrin, I'm going to do a few tests right here. We're trying to see what happened during the procedure."

I nodded in agreement, showing him that I understood what he was saying to me.

I saw him pull out what looked like a bristle brush and scrape it across the bottom of my right foot. Quickly, my reflexes retracted my foot away from the negative stimulus it was receiving. He did it once again, and I had the same reaction to the pain. Then he left. I snatched my foot away as I stared above, staring strong enough to burn a hole into the ceiling, recalling everything that had happened.

"Kerrin, squeeze my fingers." I hadn't even noticed that he was standing at the head of my bed now. I felt his two fingers firmly planted in the palm of my right hand. "Squeeze, Kerrin!" I followed the doctor's orders and squeezed as hard as I could. As he walked to my left side, I was focused on the expressions on everyone's faces. "With your left hand, squeeze my fingers." Although I thought Dr. Vaughn was a phenomenal doctor, I also thought that he could have also been a great drill sergeant, considering the way he would firmly bark orders at his patients when he needed them to do something. I kept hearing him say it over and over, "Squeeze, Kerrin, squeeze!" I was squeezing as hard as I possibly could, until . . . until I actually looked at what everyone else was looking at. Everyone else was looking at my left hand, which was NOT moving. I was confused; now it felt like I was in a dreamlike state, and the reality of the situation surely hadn't sunken in by this point. I looked up at my doctor, who was yelling at me for answers, but I said nothing. I looked at the other doctor, who was again scraping my foot; I realized that no matter how many times I had been snatching my left foot away, it wasn't actually moving—I was only snatching it away in my mind.

"Let's get her down to radiology; we need a CT scan and an MRI of the brain. Let's go, damn it!" I could see that my doctor was scared, which sent me into sheer panic. I was even more scared because he was scared, and it's quite unusual to see doctors show fear in their eyes, even when a patient is dying. As they finished the last lab test I was put into an observation room near the emergency room. My former director of nursing, who I used to refer to as "Bossy Lady," stayed beside me, explaining to me what was going on, and what I didn't understand.

She and I always made a great two-woman team when we worked together. She was far more than a boss to me then and was being far more than a nurse to me now. I was comforted for that brief moment. She held my hand as she learned over to hug me.

"They're transferring you to ICU downtown, I'll be there in the morning," she whispered into my ear. I whispered back, "Okay."

My visitor, who was also my girlfriend, entered the room. I guess an introduction was in order since it probably looked a bit odd seeing a nurse and a patient bonding in that way. As the two women acknowledged each other, I couldn't help but notice them looking at each other the way women do when they feel threatened. Their eyes were scrolling top to bottom and then back up. Both were tall, very tall, five feet eleven inches, and both were very thin, with long hair. They could have actually passed for sisters. Although I introduced them, I don't believe either said hello. They both assumed who the other one was, and it was obvious that they were sizing each other up, which made the situation uncomfortable for everyone involved.

As I explained to my girlfriend everything I had been told, she cut me off and said she already knew. She cried. I refused to cry. I consoled her. A few minutes later, a physician came into the room to speak with me. I gave her my permission that my visitor could stay and she proceeded to stay.

"We believe you suffered a stroke during the procedure and the results of that stroke have left you paralyzed on the entire left side of your body. In order to reverse the stroke we need to give you a medication called alteplase to bust the clot up, but we need to do it now. I do not need to tell you, however, that the largest complication of this medication is that it may cause a hemorrhage of the brain, which may result in death."

Shaken by what I had just heard, I closed my eyes and asked if any of the tests had confirmed that I actually had a stroke or if it was simply the doctor's best guess. The doctor replied, "No, but it may be too soon to show up. But I need your decision now. We don't have a lot of time."

I repeated what I already knew. "You're asking me to chose between being paralyzed and hemorrhaging at the brain, which could kill me?" I started to cry for the first time. *I'm going to be paralyzed or dead because I ate a god damn grape*, I thought. I continued crying for what felt like an eternity. I knew after this, I would never cry again. The patient, caring doctor let me cry for a moment before I answered her, understanding that this news had just changed the rest of my life. Finally, I answered her, "I will take paralysis. I am choosing to decline the medication."

As they transferred me downtown to the ICU of their parent hospital, I couldn't help but to continue thinking about the waitress as she had sat the first plate in front of me. I thought about what kind of patient I would be for the rest of my life, what kind of nurses I would have for the rest of my life; hopefully, nurses like myself. Then, I started praying that this whole left-sided paralysis was a test, and only a test. Today, this is my testament. I can walk. I can use my entire left side. I can still be the nurse that I am, the nurse I would always want.

Missed Diagnosis

Every nurse that I know of at some point has had the privilege or punishment of acting as a triage nurse at home. At any given moment, you get a phone call from a family member, family friend, friend of family, and even a friend of a friend that needs your nursing expertise. I've grown quite accustomed over the years to these calls. The infamous questions usually go something like, "What does it mean if my leg hurts?" or, "What should I do about my stomach pains?" or I've even been asked, "Every time I touch my stomach there's pain; what should I do?"

Most of the time, my answers are simple, yet effective. I begin by analyzing the symptoms, followed by me blurting out a few possible diagnoses based on those symptoms. I then advise them of the best way to effectively present that information to their doctor. I don't mind offering my professional advice; however, nurses are only human, and every human has their boiling point. When you get tired of being a nurse at work only to do the same thing when you arrive home, I sometimes start to blurt out answers insinuating frustration, and the replies are typically, "I don't know why it hurts; there could be one hundred reasons why your stomach hurts. If it hurts when you touch it, don't touch it!"

Often times, we nurses would simply like to punch out from work and simply be punched out! Don't get me wrong, these same nurses (including myself) mentally diagnose and second treat perfect strangers all the time. I remember looking at an overweight woman standing in line at the grocery store. She looked like she had used her last breath to make it to the checkout counter. Her legs were swollen. Her shoes were stuffed with swollen feet. Before I noticed the large goiter in her neck and the bulging eyeballs on her face, I noticed the all-pork, all-sugar-fortified diet that she had spread all over the conveyor belt. It's like nursing trivia. For those of you who are nurses, you've already diagnosed her with congestive heart failure (left sided), dyspnea on exertion hyper/hypothyroidism, and possibly diabetes. We nurses even go as far as to order labs and medications in our head that we think she needs. "Let's do on HG AIC, CMP, TSH, T3, T4, Uptake, Urinalysis; let's check for ketones." Finally, we guess that she's noncompliant with her medications but probably has prescriptions for Lasix, potassium, Levothroid, metformin, or insulin, Lipitor for her probably high cholesterol, Plavix to prevent blood clots, and probably the most desired drug on the planet, (no, not marijuana) but Norco (hydrocodone). Those would be my guesses, anyway.

Why do we voluntarily work off the clock, you ask? I don't know. I'm guessing that nursing is probably one of those professions that you simply cannot ever completely leave your work at work. At some point, everyone needs medical attention, and when your friends and family as well as perfect strangers need help, you cannot help but offer your professional advice and assistance. With all that being said, I, too, enjoy nursing trivia. Diagnosing people in public and trying to guess what's wrong with perfect strangers, yep, that's what we do..I used to pride myself on how sharp I was at detecting pain based on facial grimaces on comatose patients, detecting UTIs with patients too demented to know who they are and where they're at. Again, trivia—I love it, and I always have, until . . . until I missed the diagnosis that would change my life forever.

Anyone and everyone who has ever truly gotten to know me knew that my granny (Big D) meant the world to me. We were best friends. We were golden girls. We were partners in crime, despite our age difference. We did bingo at midnights, Pokeno on Sundays, and ran errands throughout the week together, side by side. She would call me at work to come and get bingo money so that she could go to Potowatomi Bingo with her friends throughout the week. I thought it was cute, and I didn't mind a bit. I was glad I could give it to her. Forty dollars was a small price for a big smile from my Granny. One hundred dollars was a small price, too, and that's also what I paid for a smile if she came up to my job on a day that I didn't have change. I never got change back when I gave her a one-hundred-dollar bill, but it was okay. I just figured I was paying for the next two week's smiles in advance. At seventy-two years young, she lived alone in her own house. She was a volunteer at PAEC (Provision Area for Exceptional Children), where her job title was "Classroom Grandma for Developmentally Disabled Children." She wiped noses, brushed hair, resewed buttons on zipped jackets, and even changed diapers on older kids who were incontinent. She loved her job. She loved those kids. They, too, were her grandkids.

That was my granny. That was Big D.

She had a smile that would light up a midnight sky and one dimple on her left cheek that seemed to sparkle when anyone looked at it. Most women her age have a crown of gray hair, a wheelchair or walker, and a prescription list as long as their grocery list—not my granny. She had no prescriptions for any medications, and her extremely long hair (due to her Indian heritage) shimmered; the long, silver strands resembled Christmas tinsel. Her wheelchair was a clean, well-kept, silver Cadillac that she drove everywhere.

That was my granny. That was Big D.

On September 11, 2003, I had talked on the phone to some old coworkers on a group call until two in the morning. It was then that I realized that I hadn't called my granny to tell her good night—something I did religiously. I contemplated calling her, thinking maybe she was getting in from a midnight bingo game. *Nah, I'll call her tomorrow when she's off work and let her know I'll be there Saturday morning, like always,* I thought to myself.

On Friday, September 12, I went to the hospital for my second shift. There was nothing unusual at all about the day. Relieved that the day went by kind of fast, I enjoyed my ride home and looked forward to being off of work for the weekend. I rarely ever enjoyed my ride home, but I did this time because I was the passenger and not the driver (Thanks YG!). The shoptalk on the ride home was suddenly interrupted by my cell phone ringing. I looked at it and smiled, as I always welcomed my sister Kim's phone calls.

The call went as follows:

Me: "Hello?"

Kim: "Hey, have you talked to Mom?"

Me: "No."

Kim: "Have you talked to Aunt Merl?"

Me: "No, talk to them about what?"

Kim: (crying) "You don't know, do you?"

Me: (terrified) "KNOW WHAT?!?!?!"

Kim: "Granny died."

Me: (Silence. In shock. Angry at God.)

One minute later, I was still in shock. I was empty, hollow. I, too, was dead. In a fit of rage, angry at the hands of God, I cried out from a bottomless pit that now sat where my heart used to be. I finally brought myself to speak.

Me: "What happened?!"

Kim: "She just sat at home and died while smoking a cigarette."

At this point, I said nothing. I hung up the phone on my sister, Kim. I asked my friend YG to drive me to my granny's house. I don't know why I wanted to go, but I did, and like a good friend, she took me. A week later, our family was still paralyzed. What could have happened? As we packed and loaded the last box on her donated belongings, a voice filled the air. It was one of my granny's longtime friends who was helping us pack. She went on to say:

"It was three years ago that your granny swore me to secrecy. She told me to never tell anyone, especially not her family. Five years ago, your Granny found out she had cancer of the bowel. She said she didn't want chemo or radiation. She didn't want to spend her last years in and out of the hospital. She said whatever God gave her, she would take it with her. She even told me a year ago that she had bought a new mattress because she woke up in a pool of blood. I wasn't going to say anything, but I felt so bad because everybody keeps asking why?"

There was an awkward silence. Nobody said anything. We were simply lefty. If ever there was a time I considered hanging up my stethoscope, it was then. How did this happen? How did she suffer for three years and I didn't notice one sign of one symptom? Nothing! Why? Ninety percent of my job requires me to see, observe, the obvious and the not so obvious, to notice what was missed, to listen to what others can't hear, but I didn't. I missed it. I missed every sign and every symptom. I failed. I failed me, and I failed her. I saw the woman at the checkout once and I could see everything. I had seen my granny every other day for thirty-three years and saw nothing. Why? I still don't know the answer to this question, but I think, hope, and pray that I've stopped punishing myself.

What's the lesson behind my loss? I don't know if there is one. I know that I saw silver and gold each time that I saw my granny. I saw an angel of a grandmother sent from Heaven especially for me. I saw a golden sun, no matter what color the sky was when I saw her. Every visit was magical. I saw what I wanted to see. Maybe the signs really didn't show. Maybe I was blinded by her radiance. Maybe she did her best to hide them. My last guess, which makes the most sense, and is probably the only reason I was able to pick up the pieces of my shattered life after, was the following: I saw ONLY what she wanted me to see, because that was Granny, that was Big D.

The End

Epilogue

As the tale of my intriguing dream comes to a culmination, I cannot help but to reflect upon everything that I have seen and experienced throughout my career. I went into the field of nursing thinking it was going to be a cakewalk: an easy but respectable profession. I was very wrong. Let it be known—there is nothing easy about dealing with dying people or dealing with the families of dying people. There's nothing easy about making decisions that could either save a life or even end a life. As for being a respectable profession, it is, but on a daily basis nurses are disrespected on so many levels. Being employed in healthcare makes me more grateful for and appreciative of what God has blessed me with in my personal life. It encourages me to value my relationships with family and the time we spend together. I thank GOD for all that he has done, and all that he has given me and for the time he has allowed me to have it. I also know first hand that what HE may giveth, he may taketh away. I've seen for myself from working in this field and life in general that joy, pain, and even life itself can be gone in an instant. And when it's gone, it's gone. Life is fragile, and working in this field is an everyday reminder of just how fragile life is.

I've seen people die in front of me!

I've seen people take their last breaths while I held their hand, providing a support structure so strong you wouldn't believe it.

I've seen things so traumatic I cannot even write them down in this book. I've sat beside patients and listened to them beg me to end their suffering by ending their life. A patient once said to me, "If you hit a kitten in the middle of the road and you saw it squirming out of control and covered in blood, would you look through your rearview mirror at it and keep driving until it was out of sight, or would you get out of your car to help it?" The patient went on to say that, assuming you got out of the car to help it, and saw that the little creature couldn't be saved, would you let him live and suffer until the next car came along and ran his almost-lifeless body over, or do you end his suffering now to prevent further suffering? I didn't know the answer then, and I don't know the answer now. I just know that I pay very close attention to any animals, especially kittens, when they're crossing the street. Good or bad, challenging or not, I usually find a way to come out of the situation smarter, stronger, and braver than before.

There are some specific qualities and attributes that I have that make being KJ easier, attributes that cannot be taught in school—and the sad reality is that many nurses (the majority, in fact) do not possess these attributes nor are they interested in having these great attributes. There are thousands upon thousands of very brilliant nurses practicing in the US that memorized every definition of every medical condition under the sun while they were in nursing school. They can diagnose patients even better than most doctors, too. They know all the symptoms of so many common illnesses and exactly how to treat them. Well . . . that is great, but what those aforementioned nurses do NOT have is compassion. They have no heart, and seeing a patient dying right in front of them does not have the same effect on them as it does on me. I have a big heart. I have a monumental amount of compassion. When I see a sickly patient on their deathbed, I look at them as if they were my mother, my father, my sister, or even my son. I can't help but see them that way. It makes me sick to think that some of those sick patients are not getting the very best care and the very best bedside manner in the business. Working in the medical field is not just scientifically and medically being able to treat patients, it's about having heart and compassion and being able to relate to these patients. That's what makes a great nurse. That's what makes a great person.

I am strong. I am a nurse with heart and passion. I am the nurse I would want if I were dying.

I am KJ.

Acknowledgements

I want to sincerely thank the following nursing managers:

Dr. Brenda Davis, Cinnamon Bell-Williams, Tania Thomas, (late) Dee McCollough, Fred Green, Angelina Miller, Rosie Bradley, Kathleen Mullaghy, Dorrie Seyfried-Mills, Sandra Patrick, Henry Ecker, Ellen Gaeto, Terri Karr, Lisa Subaric, and (late) Pat Benda.

The following nurses:

Anna L Jackson, Gislesa Adejola, Georgia Stewart, Thelma Joryman, Renia Bowman, Jackie Maeweather, (late) Marion Stepter, Catece Sanders, Linda Compton, Donzetta Dorsey, Jessica Bell, Latasha Robateau, Yolanda Brown, Georgia Stewart, Beverly Thomas, Jennice Lesure, (late) Karen Whitemon, Karen Whittaker, Karen Macadamia, Karen Merrell, Doris Russell, Marilyn White, Mary Rodriguez, Al Williams, Deatra Howard, (late) Theresa Smith, Melinda Perkins, (late) Tema Lyons, Genesis White, Michelle Rondez, Deidre Livingston, Sabrina Elmore, Temeka Ollie, Cherval Izimah Newsome, Roslyn Ellis, Shalese McClain, Montez Stockley, Veeda Richey, Elizabeth Kyler, Cynthia Misius, Diane Haywood, Evelyn Talon, Janet Tucker and Carmen N. Luckett.

And last but never least, the following CNAs:

Mattie Davis, Arleshia Tubbs, Alexis Parks, Ola Balogun, Emma Smith, Regina Moon, Tijuana Walker, Lisa Holloway, Jennice Lesure, Pamela Williams, Bluette, Steffon Funes, Mary Fonville, Linda Thomas, Denise Birchfield, Teresa Johnson, Coretta Goss-Simmons, Desiree Smith, Whitney Walker, Nicole Moore, Sheena Sanders, Sharon Lynn Hicks, Shavon Smith,, Elnora Holman, Thyler, Cynthia Evans, Barbara Feemster, Aisha Caffey Pat Prather, Reetta Miller, Marche Wallace, Jason James and JR Tuel.

And of course, the best nurse and doctor on the planet: Nurse Blanca and Dr. Tatum.

www.ingramcontent.com/pod-product-compliance
Lightning Source LLC
Chambersburg PA
CBHW021545200526
45163CB00015B/2007